Dr. Susan's Solutions: Pregnancy

Copyright © 2013 by Susan M. Lark, M.D.

Womens Wellness Publishing, LLC
www.womenswellnesspublishing.com
www.facebook.com/wwpublishing

Mention of specific companies or products in this book does not suggest endorsement by the author or publisher. Internet addresses and telephone numbers for resources provided in this book were accurate at the time it went to press.

Cover design by Rebecca Rose

ISBN 978-1-940188-03-4

Note: The information in this book is meant to complement the advice and guidance of your physician, not replace it. It is very important that women who have medical problems be evaluated by a physician. If you are under the care of a physician, you should discuss any major changes in your regimen with him or her. Because this is a book and not a medical consultation, keep in mind that the information presented here may not apply in your particular case. In view of individual medical requirements, new research, and government regulations, it is the responsibility of the reader to validate health practices and treatments with a physician or health service.

Acknowledgements

I want to give a huge thanks to my amazing editors Kendra Chun and Sandra K. Friend for their incredibly helpful assistance with putting this book together. I also greatly appreciate my fantastic Creative Director, Rebecca Richards, as well as Letitia Truslow, my wonderful Director of Media Relations. I enjoyed working with all of them and found their help indispensable in creating this exceptional book for women.

Table of Contents

1

Our Female Sex Hormone Production Starts with Pregnenolone

While estrogen and progesterone play the starring roles as our main female hormones, there is another hormone called pregnenolone that is equally important to our hormonal health.

Yet, it's very possible that you have never heard of pregnenolone, because it is rarely prescribed, or even discussed, by conventional physicians. However, it is the most important of the five primary sex hormones, as it plays a pivotal role in the production of all the others. As the "mother hormone" or precursor to all the major sex hormones, pregnenolone has a widespread effect throughout your entire body.

However, pregnenolone does far more than simply act as a precursor to the other sex hormones. In animal and human studies, as well as decades of clinical use, pregnenolone has been shown to relieve symptoms of PMS and support hormonal health of women during the menopause transition.

It also helps to heal a myriad of hormone-related conditions, like memory loss, rheumatoid arthritis, and other autoimmune diseases that occur much more commonly after menopause.

It also increases energy, improves cognitive function, and stabilizes moods. Other studies suggest that pregnenolone may be useful in reducing symptoms due to inflammation (which may explain why it is beneficial for treating rheumatoid arthritis), spinal-cord injuries, and possibly Alzheimer's disease.

Pregnenolone was first synthesized in Germany in 1934, and by the 1940's, researchers had begun to study its many uses, including reducing fatigue, increasing physical and mental endurance, and treating various inflammatory conditions. However, this research came to a halt in the 1950's when synthetic cortisone became the therapy of choice for such diseases as rheumatoid arthritis.

Cortisone relieved symptoms quickly, but pregnenolone sometimes required weeks to produce results. Furthermore, synthetic cortisone could be patented, turning it into a highly lucrative drug, so pharmaceutical companies were far more motivated to develop cortisone as a product, and research on pregnenolone was abandoned.

Subsequently, patients on cortisone began to suffer its harmful side effects, including a weakening of the immune system and a deterioration of bone mass leading to osteoporosis. Unfortunately, by the time these side effects were fully known, cortisone was established as a widely accepted treatment, and pregnenolone therapy, although known to be non-toxic, was forgotten.

Thankfully, pregnenolone is again being studied, thanks to the widespread, renewed interest in natural therapies. Researchers are investigating pregnenolone in relation to a wide range of topics, including memory, mood, enzyme activity, joint function, premenstrual syndrome, and the aging process. Given the exciting results of these studies, the potential benefits that pregnenolone can provide in the area of health deserves greater attention

I have written this book to share with you the great benefits that pregnenolone has on health, including many common health issues that you may personally be suffering from and looking for solutions. I will be sharing with you essential information on how to support the production of pregnenolone through the use of safe and effective all natural therapies as well as bioidentical pregnenolone replacement therapy. I have also included on the following page a chart of its many peak performance and health benefits that you may find helpful.

Benefits of Pregnenolone

Peak-Performance Benefits

- Increased physical vitality and stamina
- Enhanced mental clarity and acuity
- Increased ability to get along with other people (balances mood)

Health Benefits

- Helps to lessen symptoms of arthritis and other autoimmune diseases
- Useful in speeding recovery from spinal cord injuries
- Helpful in the treatment of Alzheimer's disease
- Helpful in the treatment of multiple sclerosis
- Helps treat PMS and perimenopause symptoms
- Treat insomnia

2

The Chemistry of Pregnenolone

In this chapter, I share with you how pregnenolone is produced within the body and how we become deficient in this essential hormone.

Pregnenolone is made primarily in the adrenal glands, but it is also produced in the cells of the liver, skin, ovaries, and brain. It is manufactured in the mitochondria, the energy-producing factories of the cells. In the mitochondria, nutrients from your diet are converted into usable energy, and cholesterol is converted into pregnenolone. The pituitary gland regulates the amount of pregnenolone produced. A study published in the *Journal of Steroid Biochemistry and Molecular Biology* found that pregnenolone accumulates in the brain, independent of sources in other areas of the body. This may have great significance, given the beneficial effects that pregnenolone seems to have on maintaining physical energy as well as stabilizing mood.

Not only pregnenolone, but all of our sex hormones, including estrogen and progesterone, are produced through a series of chemical reactions, beginning with cholesterol. Of the total cholesterol in your body, about 75 percent is produced in your liver. The remaining 25 percent is supplied in the diet by foods such as meat and dairy products. On average, a person's body contains about one-third of a pound of cholesterol (150 g), mostly as a component of cell membranes. There is also about seven grams of cholesterol that circulates in the blood.

Cholesterol is first converted into pregnenolone because it is the precursor to all the other sex hormones. Because of its precursor role, pregnenolone is considered the mother sex hormone, thus inspiring its name. Pregnenolone is then converted into a variety of other hormones, following two pathways.

By one route, pregnenolone leads to DHEA, which is then converted into testosterone and subsequently estrogen. This pathway is operative in women during the first half of the menstrual cycle, when estrogen is the dominant hormone. In the second pathway, pregnenolone is converted into progesterone. The progesterone is then converted into testosterone and, finally, into estrogen. In females, this second pathway predominates during the second half of the menstrual cycle, when progesterone and estrogen are dominant.

Although much of the body's pregnenolone is converted into other sex hormones, a certain portion of it remains unchanged and can produce a variety of beneficial effects on your health. In fact, a study published in the *Journal of Steroid Biochemistry and Molecular Biology* found that pregnenolone accumulates in the brain, independent of sources in other areas of the body. This reinforces the beneficial effects that pregnenolone seems to have on maintaining physical energy as well as stabilizing mood.

How Health and Lifestyle Affect Pregnenolone Levels

A variety of factors can decrease pregnenolone production. In particular, stress and disease can lower levels of pregnenolone throughout the body and in specific tissues, as noted in an article published in *Biochemical Pharmacology*.

Pregnenolone production also naturally decreases with age. Blood serum levels of this essential hormone can drop as much as 60% between ages 35 and 75. Obviously, as pregnenolone levels diminish, the production of all the other sex hormones arising from pregnenolone also declines. For women, much of this decline occurs with the onset of menopause. It is at this time and the years following the change that women begin to suffer from many different health issues and symptoms related to pregnenolone deficiency.

In order to maintain adequate production of pregnenolone, many systems of the body must function properly. Good digestion is required so that hormone precursors such as amino acids (the smallest units of digested protein), protein fragments, and fat molecules can be absorbed and enter the system.

Liver health also is important for pregnenolone production. When liver enzyme systems are impaired and the detoxification function is inadequate, hormone production can be affected. For instance, poor liver function can prevent the conversion of pregnenolone into DHEA. Your cholesterol profile is another factor in pregnenolone production. When the level of HDL ("good" high-density lipoproteins) is low, because it is a carrier molecule for hormones, pregnenolone production can become blocked.

In the next few chapters, I will be focusing on the many peak performance and health benefits that optimal pregnenolone levels provide to our bodies and minds.

3

Pregnenolone and Peak Performance

Although much of the body's pregnenolone is converted into other sex hormones, a certain portion of it remains unchanged and can produce a variety of effects on both health and performance.

Pregnenolone has a wide range of benefits in helping to ensure that the quality of our lives remains positive and enjoyable. For example, research studies have demonstrated that pregnenolone plays a role in increasing physical stamina and productivity when a person is working under stress. Pregnenolone can increase a person's productivity on the job.

This essential hormone improves leisure skills that require spatial thought, such as playing bridge or figuring out how to repair a dining room table. It also enhances mental acuity, concentration, and memory. An additional benefit of pregnenolone is that it has also been found to stabilize mood, thereby benefiting social relationships.

Supplementing with this hormone may be of great benefit for those individuals who want to improve performance as well as for older women, whose body's production of pregnenolone is diminishing.

In this chapter, I describe these exciting peak performance traits that are supported by an optimal supply of pregnenolone.

Physical Vitality and Stamina

In today's busy work environment, many women are experiencing a great deal of stress around the need to not only maintain a high level of energy, but also their productivity to do the very best they can with their assigned tasks. This, on top of all the other demands that women face in terms of caring for their homes and families, means that the ability to be energetic and revitalized is crucial. Research done many years ago suggests that pregnenolone can be a real help to the hundreds of thousands of women who are exceedingly busy and perhaps overwhelmed. Let's spend some time reviewing these amazing studies

Several breakthrough research studies done on pregnenolone in the 1940s have major implications for its use in maintaining physical energy and enhancing productivity. These studies were done to see if pregnenolone could improve performance and productivity among people performing complex tasks and/or operating under stressful conditions.

According to the studies, pregnenolone improved productivity under all of these conditions. Even though this research was conducted as part of the war effort and has been largely ignored for over sixty years, its implications are relevant for today's high-stress work environment.

Researchers conducted several experiments using pregnenolone in the 1940s, as reported in a 1944 article in *Aviation Medicine*. In one experiment, fourteen volunteers were trained to operate a machine designed to simulate airplane flight. The goal of the exercise was to operate the equipment properly in order to avoid obstacles and prevent crashes. Of the volunteers, seven were pilots, while the others had no flying experience. These volunteers were tested for their flying ability many times over several weeks.

Before each test, a volunteer was either given a 50 mg capsule of pregnenolone or left untreated. The results of this test showed that pregnenolone improved performance for all the volunteers. The pilots participating in the experiment also reported that their actual flying on the job improved and that they felt less tired when taking the hormone.

In another experiment reported in the same article, the researchers measured levels of a stress hormone (17-ketosteroid) in the urine of pilots. The amount of

17-ketosteroid normally increased in direct relation to the number of flights completed by the pilots. However, pilots taking pregnenolone had only half the increase in stress hormone excretion as compared with pilots not receiving pregnenolone.

Based on these results, the researchers suggested that pregnenolone can help sustain performance over a period of time. This could benefit anyone who must work long hours and perform tasks that require coordinated mental and physical activity.

The same research team conducted three other experiments, in a review article in *Biochemical Pharmacology*, in which they gave pregnenolone to three groups of skilled workers: leather cutters, lathe operators, and optical workers. The benefits of pregnenolone were assessed by monitoring units of work produced, wastage of material, and number of flaws in the finished product.

They found that when workers received a fixed wage and the work was stress-free, pregnenolone had no effect on productivity. But when workers were paid by the piece and worked under pressure, pregnenolone was associated with an increased output above their usual levels.

Given the high amount of stress in the contemporary workplace, having a sufficient amount of pregnenolone appears to be essential for peak performance.

Of particular interest in this study is that some of the volunteers taking pregnenolone also reported a sense of well-being and felt better able to cope with the requirements of their jobs.

This research is as compelling and exciting in today's work environment as it was during World War II. In many ways the demands on employees are as strenuous today as they were during that period. The prevailing reality of today's business world is that of an economic war whose objectives are for constantly higher productivity with resultant lower costs.

Most people work under constant stress, doing high precision work. Think of technicians producing computer chips under sterile conditions or surgeons performing microscopic laser surgery. The requirements and complexity of modern economic life are extraordinarily stringent. Food and nutritional products must be processed and delivered free of disease causing microorganisms, products must arrive at retailers at almost the same time the sale is made, and airplanes must operate perfectly. All of this economic complexity requires precision and great concentration.

The stresses are found throughout the economy, from automobile and computer manufacture and repair to people performing stressful mental jobs such as physicians, accountants, and book editors. Many professions require after-hours reading just to keep up with new developments in the field. Given these stresses and the fact that the population is aging, it is exciting to know that pregnenolone can support productivity and stress, especially after midlife in women when the body's natural production begins to decline.

Mental Clarity and Acuity

Pregnenolone has the potential of being of great benefit to individuals who have jobs that require them to learn and retain large quantities of new information. Most of the studies on pregnenolone and memory have been done on animals; several recent human studies have confirmed pregnenolone's potential benefits in the area of cognitive function.

Researchers designed an animal study, published in the *Proceedings of the National Academy of Sciences, USA*, which assessed the effectiveness of pregnenolone in improving the memory of mice trained to avoid electric shock as they proceeded through a maze. Some of the mice were then given individual dosages of various steroid hormones, including pregnenolone, pregnenolone sulfate, DHEA, and testosterone.

One week later, the mice were again placed in the maze to test if they remembered the correct way out. While all the hormones improved memory to some extent, pregnenolone and pregnenolone sulfate had the most potent effect.

This same team of researchers conducted another experiment, published in the *Proceedings of the National Academy of Sciences, USA*, demonstraing that even remarkably small dosages of pregnenolone can improve memory.

In this study, mice were given dosages containing fewer than 150 molecules of pregnenolone sulfate, and again post training memory processes improved. The investigators injected pregnenolone into various regions of the brain, with the amygdala (a portion of the brain believed to play an important role in arousal and alertness) proving the most sensitive.

These researchers concluded that the effectiveness of pregnenolone treatment in improving memory, when given after learning trials, may indicate that the hormone has an effect on memory storage and retrieval processes.

In the arena of human cognitive research, several recent studies suggest that pregnenolone may also enhance memory in humans. Rahmawhati Sih, M.D., a specialist in geriatrics who is affiliated with Loyola University Medical School, in Chicago, conducted several trials to explore this possibility, which she presented at a meeting of the American Federation for Medical Research.

In the study, thirteen healthy older adults — five men and eight women over the age of sixty-five — were given pregnenolone in randomly assigned quantities. Dosages were 10 mg, 50 mg, 200 mg, and 500 mg. every fourteen days, volunteers received a single dose and were asked to complete a variety of memory tests. The results of this study were promising, with memory improving somewhat as the dosage increased.

In a second trial, the volunteers were again given a range of dosages between 10 and 500 mg and asked to complete a second set of memory tests. In general, the men showed more improvement in visual/spatial tasks, while the women showed improvement in verbal recall.

Dr. Sih hypothesized that the difference in these results reflects the different metabolic pathways pregnenolone follows in men and women. In males, pregnenolone metabolizes to testosterone, which is associated with visual/spatial memory, whereas in women, pregnenolone metabolizes to estrogen, which is associated with verbal recall.

While more study is needed, these trials suggest that for older persons with diminished pregnenolone production, supplementation may prove an effective memory enhancer. This is very exciting since I have had many women patients complain about a decrease in their memory and their ability to recall many different types of information. This issue becomes much more prevalent after menopause when the production of our sex hormones, including pregnenolone, becomes a major issue for women.

The Ability to Get Along with Other People

Mood is an important determinant of how well we handle our business and social relationships. When an individual is overwhelmed by feelings of either anxiety or depression, it is difficult for them to interact with other people and maintain healthy relationships. Pregnenolone's role as a mood stabilizer can help to support this performance trait.

Because pregnenolone may play an important role in stabilizing mood due to its effect on balancing nervous system function, deficiencies may lead to mood swings and irritability. This has been confirmed by fascinating research.

A study from the journal *Molecular Pharmacology* discusses the role pregnenolone plays in regulating the delicate balance between excitation and inhibition in the central nervous system. There needs to be a balance between the excitatory neurotransmitters, which increase nerve activity, and the inhibitory neurotransmitters, which decrease nerve activity. A person in the excitatory state will experience a heightened mood and feel energized. In contrast, in the inhibitory state, an individual will feel relaxed and calm.

For normal human functioning, it is important that a balance exists between these two nervous states to avoid the extremes of anxiety and depression. And pregnenolone may play an important role in maintaining that balance.

A deficiency in pregnenolone has been linked to unstable moods in patients with emotional (affective) illness. In a study published in *Biological Psychiatry*, researchers analyzed the pregnenolone present in the cerebrospinal fluid (CSF) of twenty-seven mood-disordered patients and ten healthy volunteers as a way of measuring levels of pregnenolone.

Pregnenolone normally circulates throughout the brain and spinal column and is seen as an indicator of changes in brain chemistry. The investigators found that those patients with affective illness had lower levels of pregnenolone in the CSF compared to the healthy volunteers. Levels were especially low in those patients who were depressed on the day the CSF was drawn.

Research studies estimate that about 5 to 10 percent of the population is affected by feelings of help-lessness, low self-esteem, and poor motivation. Such a state of mind can act as an emotional barrier, preventing someone from even thinking about setting goals, let alone trying to reach them. When these feelings are caused by a deficiency of brain steroid hormones, pregnenolone supplementation may potentially help.

4

Pregnenolone and Your Health

Because pregnenolone is the "mother hormone," deficiencies can have a wide-reaching effect on your health. If your levels are below normal, you can experience PMS and perimenopause symptoms and insomnia. You may also notice a worsening of serious and debilitating physical conditions such as rheumatoid arthritis, Alzheimer's disease and, spinal-cord injuries, and even multiple sclerosis. Let's look at these issues.

PMS and Perimenopause

Premenstrual syndrome (PMS) is thought to be a result of hormonal changes. Because pregnenolone is the precursor to all sex hormones, deficiencies in this vital hormone will surely disrupt the production of other key hormones, including estrogen and progesterone, which have been linked to PMS. This can lead to a whole host of PMS-related symptoms, including fluid retention and congestion, irritability, anxiety, and depression.

Connie's Story

When Connie came to see me, she was 46 years old. She had always had severe PMS symptoms, with moodiness, headaches, breast tenderness, and menstrual cramps. Although she has always had regular menstrual periods, she was now in the early stages of premenopause.

She began experiencing irregular periods and her mood swings had worsened. She was also experiencing joint pain and inflammation, and was told by her doctor that she had early signs of rheumatoid arthritis.

Connie started using pregnenolone, the precursor to progesterone, along with a very strong nutritional program, to help her deal with her PMS and premenopause symptoms.

Within a few short weeks, she began to feel significantly better. Over a period of several months, her joints became less sore, her periods were more regular, and she had an even, balanced mood.

Insomnia

Women in transition and those who have entered menopause often suffer from insomnia or poor sleep quality. In fact, it is one of the most common health issues that women suffer from, draining energy and vitality and the ability to carry out our day-to-day tasks. There is almost nothing worse than tossing and turning in bed at night, having frequent wakes ups and then getting up in the morning feeling tired and exhausted in the morning instead of refreshed and energized.

In addition to hormonal changes causing insomnia, but many women are engaged in work that causes them to be sleep deprived such as late shift nurses, emergency room doctors, hospitality industry employees, factory workers and women who frequently travel for their jobs and must travel late at night.

Research studies have shown that sleep deprivation can lower productivity through the interruption of normal biological cycles. Pregnenolone may be beneficial for those individuals whose jobs require them to work swing or late shifts.

Pregnenolone not only offers promise in improving work productivity by increasing physical energy and mental alertness, but it may also help to improve productivity and maintain energy in workers who are sleep deprived. In a study published in *Brain*

Research, twelve healthy male volunteers, aged 20 to 30, who were given pregnenolone experienced improved sleep quality and were also less likely to wake intermittently during the sleep period.

These results are particularly impressive since the effects of this study were achieved using a dosage of only 1 mg of pregnenolone, given orally before sleep. The normal range of dosage for pregnenolone is much greater, typically 5 to 50 mg per day.

Women with sleep related issues may want to consider using pregnenolone rather than prescription medication in order to get a good night's sleep on a consistent basis.

Alzheimer's Disease

A review article on pregnenolone published in *Pergamon* suggested that it may one day be proven useful in the treatment of Alzheimer's disease. This degenerative brain disease is characterized by loss of memory and other cognitive functions. The progression of the disease is believed to involve a low-grade inflammatory process that is self-perpetuating and interferes with the body's ability to repair itself.

Pregnenolone may prove to be an effective anti-inflammatory therapy for the treatment of this disease. As pregnenolone is nontoxic and readily absorbed, it has great potential as a treatment and deserves further investigation in this capacity.

Arthritis and Autoimmune Disease

Women who are deficient in pregnenolone are at higher risk for rheumatoid arthritis and other inflammatory diseases, such as systemic lupus erythematosus (an autoimmune condition), ankylosing spondylitis (a chronic inflammatory disease of the joints in the spine that causes back stiffening and pain), scleroderma (a rigidity and hardening of the skin and even fibrosis of internal organs), and psoriasis.

Let's look at rheumatoid arthritis. Early research studies suggest that pregnenolone may be effective in treating patients in the early stages of rheumatoid arthritis, lessening symptoms associated with inflammation. When your body has adequate amounts of the hormone, inflammation is kept at bay. However, if your body is deficient in pregnenolone, inflammation and its nasty sidekicks, including rheumatoid arthritis, show up. To this point, a study from the *Annals of the New York Academy of Sciences* found that people with rheumatoid arthritis have significantly depleted levels of pregnenolone (as well as DHEA-S and testosterone). Therefore, researchers have concluded that supplemental pregnenolone can help ease rheumatoid arthritis symptoms.

Another study followed the results of pregnenolone treatment of eleven patients with rheumatoid arthritis. Of these men and women, ranging in age from 34 to 65, six experienced moderate to marked improvement, and some of the others showed slight improvement. Furthermore, between the third and seventh day of therapy, patients noted a sense of well being and improved appetite. And between the fourth and eighth days, patients reported a noticeable reduction in joint pain. This improvement allowed greater joint mobility and reduced muscular atrophy. In some of the patients, there was also less swelling in the joints.

Rheumatoid arthritis is much more prevalent in women than men and the incidence of this crippling illness significantly increases after menopause. This is the time when all sex hormones, including pregnenolone, significantly decrease. Along with the other female hormones, pregnenolone replacement therapy may be very helpful for this group of women.

Other studies have also suggested that pregnenolone has potential in the treatment of other inflammatory diseases such as systemic lupus erythematosus (an autoimmune condition), ankylosing spondylitis (a chronic inflammatory disease of the joints in the spine that causes back stiffening and pain), scleroderma (a rigidity and hardening of the skin and even fibrosis of internal organs), and psoriasis.

While much more research needs to be done in this area, pregnenolone may eventually prove to be an exciting new and effective therapy for these disabling chronic conditions.

Multiple Sclerosis

Multiple sclerosis is a disease of the central nervous system involving progressive destruction of the myelin sheath surrounding the nerves. This disease commonly affects young and middle-aged adults, causing symptoms such as weakness, loss of coordination, unsteady gait, and visual deterioration.

Researchers have found that pregnenolone may play an important role, along with the female hormone progesterone, in the healing of damaged nerves. Another study, published in *Science*, confirmed these findings. This study found that when progesterone and pregnenolone were administered, myelin sheath development progressed normally. However, much more research on the use of pregnenolone as a treatment for multiple sclerosis remains to be done.

Spinal Cord Injuries

Pregnenolone is useful in reducing the inflammation that occurs at the time of accident in spinal-cord injuries. The inflammation that occurs as a result of these injuries can cause tissue damage and may even lead to permanent functional impairment and paralysis. By reducing inflammation, pregnenolone speeds recovery and helps prevent further health problems. Because so many factors are involved in recovery from a spinal-cord injury, any single therapy is usually not effective in reversing this process.

Combining pregnenolone with other therapeutic agents may lead to improved recovery from this serious health issue. This was investigated in an animal study published in the *Proceedings of the National Academy of Sciences, USA.*

In this study, investigators combined several treatments including pregnenolone; DHEA (dehydro-epiandrosterone); indomethacin (IM), an anti-inflammatory compound; and bacterial lipopoly-saccharide (LPS), a substance that stimulates cytokine secretion (cytokines are intercellular messengers that regulate many cell functions, especially those related to immunologic and inflammatory responses).

This combination of therapies was given to animals that had undergone injury. In twenty-one days after the injury, eleven of sixteen animals were able to stand and walk, four of the animals almost normally. Of all the therapies administered, the combination of IM, LPS, and pregnenolone produced notably significant improvements. This treatment was far more effective than any of the treatments given independently or in any combination of two.

5

Testing for Pregnenolone Deficiency

If you suspect that you may be deficient in pregnenolone, it is important to be evaluated for this essential hormone if you are considering replacement or supportive therapy. In this chapter, I share with you a very helpful questionnaire that I developed to help you pinpoint important areas of your health and well being in which pregnenolone may play an important role. You may want to fill out this questionnaire to determine if you want to undergo laboratory testing for your pregnenolone level.

Are You Pregnenolone Deficient?

The following checklist will give you an idea of whether you are experiencing the effects of low pregnenolone. If you answer yes to three or more of these questions, you may want to consider further evaluation and support of your pregnenolone levels.

Pregnenolone Deficiency Checklist

- ○ I have a history of PMS.
- ○ I am in perimenopause.
- ○ I am in menopause.
- ○ My sleep quality is poor; I tend to wake up intermittently during the night.
- ○ I have a negative state of mind.
- ○ I have unstable moods, am irritable, and/or tend to be depressed.
- ○ I am unable to work efficiently and effectively under stress.
- ○ I have low energy and lack stamina.
- ○ I have a poor memory.
- ○ I have poor verbal recall.
- ○ I'm at risk for Alzheimer's disease.
- ○ I have a history of autoimmune disease, including rheumatoid arthritis, systemic lupus erythematosus, ankylosing spondylitis, scleroderma, and/or psoriasis.
- ○ I have a history of multiple sclerosis.
- ○ I have a history of spinal cord injury.

If your responses suggest that your pregnenolone level may be low, then your next step is to get your hormone levels tested.

Laboratory Testing for Pregnenolone

Pregnenolone levels are assessed by measuring the amount of pregnenolone sulfate in the blood. Pregnenolone sulfate is transported more efficiently through the circulatory system because it is more water-soluble than pregnenolone.

In adult men, blood levels of pregnenolone sulfate are about 10 mcg per 100 ml. Average daily production of pregnenolone is about 14 mg a day, a relatively small amount (30,000 mg equals about one ounce). These amounts may vary significantly among individuals.

Levels of pregnenolone can be measured in the blood and the saliva. Tests can be ordered to assess the quantity present of pregnenolone, pregnenolone sulfate, and 17- hydroxy-pregnenolone. The latter is the intermediary hormone in the conversion of pregnenolone to DHEA.

Experts caution on the usefulness of such tests. There is not a lot of information on what consists of a normal reading in different age groups. It is also not known how accurately blood levels represent tissue levels of the hormone. Various tissues may also make use of pregnenolone in different ways, so that a blood reading would tell little about its eventual activity level.

Health care practitioners who place patients on pregnenolone therapy recommend especially close monitoring of levels, since taking this hormone as a supplement is somewhat new.

Ranges of Pregnenolone Levels:

Taking these questions into consideration, the following ranges for blood levels of pregnenolone are used by several labs:

Pregnenolone production in adult women:

10 to 230 ng/dl

Pregnenolone production in postmenopausal women:

5 to 100 ng/dl

If your results indicate that you are deficient in pregnenolone, or if you scored high on the checklist, help is just a few pages away. Let's take a look at the many ways you can restore your pregnenolone levels quickly and effectively, while helping to ultimately improve the production of all your sex hormones.

6

Support Your Own Production of Pregnenolone

Low levels of the mother hormone can throw all of your sex hormones out of balance. In this chapter, I'll share with you my program to help you restore and maintain proper pregnenolone levels. I'll discuss how you can restore this critical hormone at the central nervous system level, with the help of some key neurotransmitters and glandulars, as well as a few little-known herbs. You'll also discover how vital vitamins and nutrients can help to keep your pregnenolone levels in the healthy range by optimizing adrenal and ovarian function.

Let's get started!

Support Pregnenolone Production from the Central Nervous System

All sex hormone production begins in the brain, and pregnenolone is no exception. While women are surprised to learn that you can increase progesterone production through the brain or central nervous system, the truth is that all hormone production begins in the brain.

We've been traditionally taught that human beings have one brain that is divided into many different parts. But more and more research is putting the "one brain" idea to the test. In fact, it's starting to be widely accepted that the human skull actually houses not one brain, but three — the reptilian brain, the limbic brain, and the neocortical brain.

The reptilian brain is the oldest part of the brain. It controls basic bodily functions like heart rate, breathing, body temperature, hunger, and fight-or-flight responses. Basic drives and instincts, such as defending territory and keeping safe from harm, are other functions of the reptilian brain. The structures in the brain that perform these functions are the brain stem (which controls breathing, heart rate, and blood pressure) and the cerebellum (which controls movement, balance, and posture).

The limbic, or mammalian, brain developed once mammals started roaming the earth. It includes the amygdala, which controls memory and emotions; the hippocampus, which controls memories and learning; and the hypothalamus, which controls emotions (among many other things). Therefore, the limbic brain allows mammals to learn, retain memories, and show emotions.

The neocortical brain, or neocortex, is the complex maze of grey matter that surrounds the reptilian and limbic brains, and accounts for about 85 percent of brain mass. It is found in the brains of primates and humans, and is responsible for sensory perception, abstract thought, imagination, and consciousness. It also controls language, social interactions, and higher communication.

The Chemistry of the Brain

Like the three parts of the brain, there are also three key types of brain chemicals: neuropeptides, neuro-hormones, and neurotransmitters.

Neuropeptides are responsible for the cell-to-cell communication system in your body. A peptide is a short chain of amino acids connected together, and a neuropeptide is a peptide found in neural tissue. Neuropeptides are widespread in the central and peripheral nervous systems and different neuro-peptides have different excitatory or inhibitory actions.

Neuropeptides control such a diverse array of functions in the body. When they work together properly, the wonderful results in your body include elevated mood and other positive behaviors and emotions, stronger bones, better resistance to disease, glowing skin, and boosted metabolism. Conversely, if your neuropeptides function abnormally, the result can be an increased tendency towards neurological and mental disorders such as Alzheimer's disease, epilepsy, and schizophrenia.

There are several types of neuropeptides. Some of the most common include endorphins and beta-endorphins. Endorphins are opiod peptides, meaning they have morphine-like effects within the body. They produce feelings of well-being and euphoria, and a rush of endorphins can lead to feelings of exhilaration brought on by pain, danger, or stress. Endorphins also may also play a role in memory, sexual activity, and body temperature. Beta-endorphins are another form of opiod peptides, but they are stronger than endorphins. They are composed of 31 amino acids and work in the body by numbing pain, increasing relaxation, and promoting a general feeling of well-being.

While there are many hormones and hormonal interactions that occur in the brain and body, the most widely known neurohormone is melatonin. This is the hormone produced by the pineal gland, which regulates our patterns of sleep.

Neurotransmitters are naturally occurring chemicals that relay electrical messages between nerve cells throughout your body. While all three types of neurochemicals are important for hormone and overall health, neurotransmitters are particularly important for the production of sex hormones.

In the aggregate, all three types of neurochemicals help to regulate the brain's endocrine glands, specifically the hypothalamus and pituitary gland. The hypothalamus is the master endocrine gland contained within your brain that regulates your production of sex hormones, including pregnenolone. Without this system functioning properly, the production of pregnenolone and your other sex hormones is greatly impaired.

The hypothalamus produces a precursor hormone called gonadotropin releasing hormone (GnRH), which initiates the entire cascade through which pregnenolone and our other sex hormones are produced. The neurotransmitters norepinephrine, epinephrine, dopamine, and serotonin play an extremely important role in this entire process because they regulate the hypothalamus' release of GnRH. Without proper production and balance of these neurotransmitters, you cannot have proper production and even balance of the sex hormones, including the production of pregnenolone.

Neurotransmitters also support the production of hormones by the pituitary gland. These processes are supported by precursor amino acids such as tyrosine, phenylalanine, and 5-HTP. Neurotransmitters are produced by the conversion of these amino acids. This occurs in the presence of essential vitamins and minerals such as vitamin C, vitamin B6, and magnesium.

To understand this more fully, let's take a more detailed look at neurotransmitters in action.

The Key to Unlocking Hormone Production

There are two crucial neurotransmitter pathways that help to support your overall health and well-being. The first leads to the production of inhibitory neurotransmitters like serotonin and GABA. The second leads to the production of excitatory neurotransmitters such as dopamine, norepinephrine, and epinephrine, as well as glutamate.

Generally speaking, the inhibitory neurotransmitters quiet down the processes of your body, while the excitatory neurotransmitters speed them up. Thus, the brain chemicals produced through these two pathways oppose and complement one another. Within your brain, serotonin often inhibits the firing of neurons, which dampens many of your behaviors. In fact, serotonin acts as a kind of chemical restraint system.

Of all your body's chemicals, serotonin has one of the most widespread effects on the brain and physiology. It plays a key role in regulating temperature, blood pressure, blood clotting, immunity, pain, digestion, sleep, and biorhythms. Along with another inhibitory neurotransmitter, GABA (gamma aminobutyric acid), serotonin also produces a relaxing effect on your mood. Taurine, a type of amino acid, is often used in a similar fashion as these two neurotransmitters due to its therapeutic, inhibitory effects in your body.

Dopamine, norepinephrine, and epinephrine make up the excitatory neurotransmitter pathway. Glutamate is another important excitatory neurotransmitter, though it is not part of the pathway. Unlike serotonin, which has a relaxing effect on your energy and behavior, excitatory neurotransmitters energize and elevate your mood. In addition to their powerful anti-depressant effects, they support alertness, optimism, motivation, zest for life, and sex drive. Plus, the excitatory neurotransmitters are particularly important for the production of progesterone.

In order to ensure that you have adequate neurotransmitter levels for healthy hormone production, you need to supplement with key amino acids, vitamins, and minerals. All neurotransmitters are produced from amino acids found in the protein that you eat. The essential amino acid tryptophan is initially converted into an intermediary substance called 5-hydroxytryptophan (5-HTP), which is then converted into serotonin.

While tryptophan is available as a supplement and is abundant in turkey, pumpkin seeds, and almonds, I have found that 5-HTP is more effective and reliable for boosting your neurotransmitter production.

Numerous double-blind studies have shown that 5-HTP is as effective as many of the more common antidepressant drugs and is associated with fewer and much milder side effects. In addition to increasing serotonin levels, 5-HTP triggers a rise in endorphins and other neurotransmitters that are often low in cases of depression.

The excitatory neurotransmitters are derived from tyrosine, an amino acid produced from phenylalanine, another amino acid. A variety of vitamins and minerals, such as vitamin C, vitamin B6, and magnesium, act as co-factors and are necessary for the conversion of these amino acids into neurotransmitters.

To maintain proper serotonin levels, it is helpful to take 50-100 mg of 5-HTP once or twice a day, with one of the dosages taken at bedtime. Be sure to start at 50 mg and increase as necessary. If needed during the day, use carefully, as too much serotonin can interfere with your ability to drive or concentrate.

To maintain optimum dopamine levels, take 500-1,000 mg of tyrosine per day. Be sure to take in divided doses, half in the morning and half in the afternoon. Do not take in the evening, as it may interfere with sleep.

43   Pregnenolone

As I recommend with all nutritional supplements, you should start at the lower to more moderate dosage, such as 500 mg a day of tyrosine and 50 mg a day of 5-HTP. Stay on this dosage for two weeks. If you don't notice a reduction in your symptoms, gradually increase the dosage by 500 mg for tyrosine and 50 mg for 5-HTP every two weeks until you have either noticed a reduction in your symptoms or have reached the maximum dosages. I generally don't recommend going over 1,000 mg a day of tyrosine, although you may find that you need as much as 100-200 mg of 5-HTP once or even several times a day.

Additionally, be sure to use a high potency multi-vitamin or mineral nutritional supplements so that you are taking in all of the co-factors needed to produce neurotransmitters. These include vitamin C, vitamin B6, folic acid, niacin, magnesium, and copper.

Note: I strongly advise that you undertake a program to restore and properly balance your neuro-transmitter levels under the care of a complementary physician, naturopath, or nutritionist. You should also have your neurotransmitter levels tested regularly, as dosage needs for the amino acids I have described often vary from woman to woman.

Test Your Neurotransmitter Levels

State-of-the-art neurotransmitter testing is currently available and can accurately pinpoint your exact levels of these essential brain chemicals. A leader in the development of neurotransmitter testing is NeuroScience, Inc, (888-342-7272 or Neurorelief.com). They have developed sensitive testing for neuro-chemicals that can be done through your urine. The test is simple to do, non-invasive, and can be done in the privacy of your own home. In addition to NeuroScience, there are many other similar laboratories that offer neurotransmitter testing.

I would strongly recommend that you consider such testing if you suspect that you suffer from a moderate to severe neurotransmitter deficiency. Your health care provider will need to order these tests for you.

Support Pregnenolone Production in the Ovaries and Adrenals

While hormone production begins in your brain, the actual production of pregnenolone takes place primarily in your adrenals and ovaries, making it critical that you keep these glands functioning at their optimal level. To do this, I highly recommend using the following key nutrients: glandulars, beta-carotene, vitamin C, vitamin B5, zinc, and magnesium.

Glandular Therapy

Glandular therapy involves the use of purified extracts from the secretory endocrine glands of animals. Most commonly, extracts are drawn from the thyroid and adrenal glands, as well as the thymus, pituitary, pancreas, and ovaries.

In the past, most experts believed that glandulars could not be effective because the intestinal lining of a healthy person was impenetrable, and that proteins and large peptides could not breach its barrier.

However, recent evidence has shown that large macromolecules can and do pass completely intact from the intestinal tract into the bloodstream. In fact, there's further evidence to suggest that your body is able to determine which molecules it needs to absorb whole, and which can be broken down.

Both animal and human studies alike have proven this theory. In some cases, several whole proteins taken orally, including critical enzymes, have been shown to be absorbed intact into the bloodstream. Additionally, many smaller proteins and numerous hormones have also been found to be absorbed intact into the bloodstream, including thyroid, cortisone, and even insulin.

In essence, it means that the active properties of the glandulars stay active and intact, and are not destroyed in the digestive process. This is significant to the success of glandular therapy, and explains why they clearly help to restore hormone function by supporting the health of your endocrine glands themselves.

There are multi- and single-glandular systems available from companies like Standard Process — a leader in the field. However, they do require a prescription from a health care practitioner. Other good products are also available in health food stores and should be used as part of a nutritional program to support healthy menstruation.

One of the most widely used and accepted glandulars is for your adrenal glands. Whole adrenal glandular preparations are not only beneficial in treating stress and fatigue; they have been shown to possess cortisone-like properties that help treat asthma, eczema, rheumatoid arthritis, and even psoriasis. They have also been found to help restore the health and function of comprised adrenal glands.

In one research study, eight women suffering from morning sickness (nausea and vomiting) who took oral adrenal cortex extract found relief within four days. A similar study gave both injected and oral adrenal cortex extract to 202 women also suffering from morning sickness. More than 85 percent of the women completely overcame their nausea and vomiting or showed significant improvement.

Another study looked at the use of adrenal gland-ulars to treat patients with chronic fatigue and immune dysfunction syndrome (CFIDS), as well as fibromyalgia. Researchers found that 5-13 mg of an adrenal glandular preparation significantly reduced pain and discomfort. Moreover, after six to 18 months, many of the patients were able to reduce and eventually discontinue treatment, while still enjoying relief.

Clearly, glandulars work. To help support healthy pregnenolone levels, I suggest taking a good multi-glandular or single glandular product from a company like Standard Process. These could include glandulars such as adrenal, ovary, hypothalamus, and pituitary, depending on your specific needs. To boost pregnenolone production even further than the endocrine glands of the brain, you may also want to focus on adrenal and ovarian support specifically. I also highly recommend that you consider taking a whole brain glandular, if appropriate.

Boost Hormone Production With Key Nutrients
In addition to powerful glandulars, there are several important nutrients that are critical to the health of your adrenal glands and ovaries. By supporting the function of the adrenals and ovaries, these important nutrients ensure the proper production and balance of adrenal and ovarian hormones, including pregnen-olone.

Beta-carotene is the plant-based, water-soluble precursor to vitamin A. It is very abundant in the adrenal glands and is important for the healthy functioning of the ovaries. It is particularly plentiful in the corpus luteum of the ovary. After ovulation, the follicle that contained the egg that was expelled from the ovary during ovulation is then converted into a new structure called the corpus luteum. The purpose of the corpus luteum is to switch from the estrogen production, which predominates during the first half of the menstrual cycle (days 1 to 14) to the production of progesterone and estrogen during the second half of your cycle (days 15 to 28). This is called the luteinizing process. Some research studies even suggest that a proper balance between carotene and the retinal form of vitamin A is necessary for proper luteal function.

To ensure that you have adequate amounts of vitamin A (as beta-carotene) in your system, I suggest taking 25,000-50,000 IU of beta-carotene a day. You can also eat foods rich in beta-carotene, such as spinach, squash, carrots, cantaloupe, pumpkin, and sweet potatoes.

Vitamin C is very well known for its cold- and flu-fighting properties, but most people don't realize that it is an integral part of the structure and function of the adrenal glands. Your adrenals have the highest concentration of vitamin C in your entire body. These

49   Pregnenolone

glands use the vitamin to synthesize a variety of hormones and neurotransmitters, namely norepinephrine, epinephrine, and serotonin.

Furthermore, the adrenals use vitamin C to produce cortisol, which is released in times of stress. In fact, studies have shown that when you are under extreme stress, your vitamin C stores are rapidly depleted. This means that your entire body suffers from vitamin C deficiency due to acute stress, with your adrenal glands taking the biggest hit.

To be sure your adrenal glands have adequate amounts of vitamin C, take 1,000-3,000 mg of a mineral-buffered vitamin C each day, in divided doses. Also increase your consumption of vitamin C-rich foods, including citrus fruits, strawberries, peaches, broccoli, tomatoes, and spinach.

B vitamins, especially B5 (pantothenic acid), play a crucial role in adrenal function. They are critical for stress management, neurotransmitter synthesis, and hormone production and regulation. In particular, B5 is the primary nourishing nutrient of your adrenal glands. It is necessary to stimulate the adrenal glands to begin hormone production, including pregnenolone. B5 is also needed to produce glucocorticoids, including cortisol. Not surprisingly, the symptoms of vitamin B5 deficiency—fatigue, headaches, sleep issues—mimic those of adrenal exhaustion.

For proper adrenal function, be sure to take 50-100 mg of a vitamin B-complex a day, with an additional 250-500 mg of B5 daily. You can also increase your intake of foods high in B vitamins, including liver, wheat germ, whole grains, legumes, egg yolks, salmon, royal jelly, sweet potatoes, and brewer's yeast.

Zinc not only supports healthy adrenal function, but it helps to produce testosterone and progesterone. By promoting proper pregnenolone production, this essential trace mineral also helps in a variety of enzymatic functions, aids in vitamin A metabolism, and keeps your immune system strong.

To ensure that your adrenal glands have adequate amounts of zinc, I suggest taking 10-25 mg of zinc a day. You can also eat foods rich in zinc, such as oysters, pumpkin seeds, and eggs.

Magnesium is one of the basic building blocks needed by your adrenals to produce hormones. Adequate amounts of this vital mineral are also necessary to keep your adrenals balanced and functioning properly. Research has shown that low levels of magnesium can often indicate an overly stressed adrenal system. In fact, depressed and suicidal people have been found to be magnesium deficient.

You can maintain healthy adrenal function with 600-1,000 mg of magnesium a day, as well as eating foods like meat, nuts, whole grains, and dairy, all of which are high in magnesium.

Maintain Adrenal Health With Adaptogenic Herbs

Like key vitamins and minerals, adaptogenic herbs also support the adrenals, ovaries, and other endocrine glands, thereby preventing the long-term adrenal burnout and exhaustion that occurs with chronic stress. (An adaptogen is a substance that is innocuous, is able to increase resistance to a wide range of adverse physical, chemical, and biochemical factors, and promotes a normalization between extremes.) These herbs also contain a wide variety of chemicals that help the body recover more quickly from hard physical labor, athletic exertion, and even convalescence from surgery.

Rhodiola rosea was used medicinally by the ancient Greeks as far back as 100 A.D. Named for the rose-like odor of the rootstock when newly cut, Siberian healers believe that people who drink Rhodiola tea on a regular basis will have the potential to live to be more than 100 years old. And in Russia, Rhodiola has been used to diminish fatigue and increase your body's resistance to stress.

Rhodiola works to support all hormone production by easing stress and fatigue. Both destroy adrenal function and healthy sex hormone production, including pregnenolone. According to the journal *Phytomedicine*, Rhodiola is particularly effective in fighting stress-induced fatigue. In one study, researchers tested 40 male medical students during exam time to determine if the herb positively affected physical fitness, as well as mental well-being and capacity.

The students were divided into two groups and given either 50 mg of Rhodiola rosea extract or placebo twice a day for 20 days. Researchers found that those students who took the extract had a significant decrease in mental fatigue and improved psychomotor function, with a 50% improvement in neuromotor function. In addition, scores from exams taken immediately after the study showed that the extract group had an average grade of 3.47, as compared to 3.20 for the placebo group.

To ease fatigue, stress, or anxiety—all of which can play havoc with your pregnenolone production—I recommend taking 50-100 mg of Rhodiola rosea three times a day, standardized to 3 percent rosavins and 0.8 percent salidrosides. While the herb is generally considered safe, some reports have indicated that it may counteract the effects of anti-arrhythmic medications. Therefore, if you are currently taking this type of medication, I suggest you discuss the use of Rhodiola rosea with your physician.

Panax ginseng has been used in Chinese herbal medicine for more than 4,000 years. While the wild form is now rare, panax ginseng is widely cultivated. High quality ginseng improves the strength and balance of our endocrine glands, thereby supporting the production of our sex hormones, including pregnenolone. Many of the symptoms linked to pregnenolone deficiency can be decreased with the use of ginseng.

Ginseng also has a balancing, tonic effect on the systems and organs of the body involved in the stress response. It contains at least 13 different saponins, a class of chemicals found in many plants, especially legumes, which take their name from their ability to form a soap like froth when shaken with water. These compounds (triterpene glycosides) are the most pharmaceutically active constituents of ginseng. Saponins benefit hormone production, as well as cardiovascular function, immunity, and the central nervous system.

During times of stress, the saponins in the ginseng act on the hypothalamus and pituitary glands, increasing the release of adrenocorticotrophin, or ACTH (a hormone produced by the pituitary that promotes the manufacture and secretion of adrenal hormones). As a result, ginseng increases the release of adrenal cortisone and other adrenal hormones, and prevents their depletion from stress. Other substances associated with the pituitary are also released, such as endorphins. Ginseng is used to prevent adrenal atrophy, which can be a side effect of cortisone drug treatment. Ginseng's ability to support the health and function of the adrenal glands during times of stress, as well as the improved hormone health that occurs with the use of ginseng, clearly supports the production of pregnenolone itself by the adrenal glands.

In a study published in *Drugs Under Experimental and Clinical Research*, two groups of volunteers suffering from fatigue due to physical or mental stress were given nutritional supplementation over a 12-week period. One hundred sixty-three volunteers were given a multivitamin and multi mineral complex, and 338 volunteers received the same product, plus a standardized Chinese ginseng extract. Once a month, the volunteers were asked to fill out a questionnaire during a scheduled visit with a physician. This questionnaire contained 11 quest-ions that asked them to describe their current level of perceived physical energy, stamina, sense of well-being, libido, and quality of sleep.

While both groups experienced similar improvement in their quality of life by the second visit, the group using the ginseng extract almost doubled their improvement, based on their responses, by the third and fourth visits. Thus, ginseng, when added to a multivitamin and multi mineral complex, appears to improve many factors of well-being in individuals experiencing significant physical and emotional stress.

There is also evidence that ACTH (the hormone that stimulates the adrenal cortex) and adrenal hormones, which ginseng stimulates, are known to bind to brain tissue, increasing mental activity during stress.

For maximum benefit, take a high quality suplement, an extract of the main root of a plant that is six to eight years old, standardized for ginsenoside content and ratio. Companies manufacturing ginseng products may mention the age of the plants used in their products as a testimony to their products' quality. Take a 100 mg capsule twice a day. If this is too stimulating, especially before bedtime, take the second dose mid-afternoon, or take only the morning dose. Women using ginseng should purchase either Chinese or American ginseng that is better for the female body. Avoid Korean Red Ginseng that is better suited for men and too heating for the female body.

The documented side effects of ginseng include nervousness, hypertension, morning diarrhea, skin problems, insomnia, and euphoria. It is important that a person taking ginseng monitor themselves for these symptoms.

Siberian ginseng (Eleutherococcus senticosus) is part of the same family as panax ginseng, but the exact composition differs considerably. The most pharmacologically active constituents in Siberian ginseng are eleutherosides, some of which are similar in structure to the saponins contained in Asian ginseng. Siberian ginseng has been used in Asia for nearly 2,000 years to combat fatigue and increase endurance. The medicinal properties of this plant have been studied in Russia, with a number of clinical and experimental studies demonstrating that eleutherosides are adaptogenic, increasing resistance to stress and fatigue.

According to a review of clinical trials of more than 2,100 healthy human subjects, ranging in age from 19 to 72, published in *Economic Medicinal Plant Research*, Siberian ginseng reduces activation of the adrenal cortex in response to stress, an action useful in the alarm stage of the fight-or-flight response. It also helps lower blood pressure. In this same study, data indicated that the eleutherosides increased the subjects' ability to withstand adverse physical conditions including heat, noise, motion, an increase in workload, and exercise. There was also improved quality of work under stressful work conditions and improved athletic performance.

57   Pregnenolone

Herbalists have also long prescribed Siberian ginseng for chronic-fatigue syndrome. One way in which ginseng may be effective in this capacity is through its ability to facilitate the conversion of fat into energy, in both intense and moderate physical activity, sparing carbohydrates, and postponing the point at which a person may "hit the wall." This occurs when stored glucose is depleted and can no longer serve as a source of energy.

Siberian ginseng is also used to treat a variety of psychological disturbances, including insomnia, hypochondriasis, and various neuroses. The reason Siberian ginseng is effective may be its ability to balance stress hormones from the adrenals and neurotransmitters such as epinephrine, serotonin, and dopamine, all of which support healthy hormone production by the adrenal glands and ovaries, including pregnenolone.

Though Siberian ginseng has virtually no toxicity, individuals with fever, hypertonic crisis, or myocardial infarction are advised not to use it. A standard dosage of the fluid extract (33 percent ethanol) ranges from 3-5 ml, three times a day, for periods of up to 60 consecutive days. An equivalent dosage of dry powdered extract (containing at least one percent eleutheroside F) is 100-200 mg three times a day. Take in multiple-dose regimens with two to three weeks between courses.

Take Care When Choosing Ginseng

I have had a number of patients over the years who have bought inexpensive ginseng, either as a root or in capsule form, expecting miraculous results, given ginseng's venerable reputation. Unfortunately, these cheaper grades of ginseng rarely, if ever, deliver the punch that individuals expect — that is, the chemical equivalent of an auxiliary set of adrenal glands, testicles, or ovaries.

I have seen some remarkable results with high-grade ginseng purchased from reputable Chinese pharmacists that sell top-of-the-line herbs or American companies selling herbs of equivalent quality. Given that the potency of the therapeutic chemicals takes many years to develop within the ginseng root, it is no surprise that with ginseng, you get what you pay for. If you have a serious interest in using ginseng, for its adaptogenic properties, I strongly suggest that you search out the reputable dealers.

7

The Benefits of Bioidentical Pregnenolone

Bioidentical pregnenolone replacement therapy can be a very useful treatment option for women wanting to supplement their own levels of this essential hormone. Bioidentical pregnenolone is available over the counter and is sold in pharmacies and natural-food stores. It can also be ordered by a physician from a compounding pharmacy.

Pregnenolone is often made from either soy or the Mexican wild yam, both of which belong to the Dioscorea species. (The Mexican wild yam is not related to the yams and sweet potatoes found in the supermarket, so eating these will not increase hormone levels.)

The active steroid compound used in manufacture is diosgenin, which has a chemical structure closely related to the structure of the hormones in our own body. To make pregnenolone, diosgenin must be converted in a laboratory. For this reason, when purchasing pregnenolone, it is important to note if the container specifically states that the product contains pregnenolone, rather than just an un-processed extract of wild yam.

Many people take pregnenolone rather than DHEA, which is also a powerful precursor hormone, because a much lower dose of pregnenolone can enhance the central nervous system function. Other advantages of pregnenolone are that it has more potent anti-inflammatory effects and is less likely than DHEA to cause side effects such as skin problems and facial hair.

Pregnenolone is available as an oral pill or capsule, in a micronized form, as a sublingual tablet, as an ointment or cream, and in a liposome-based oral spray. The degree to which pregnenolone is absorbed and the amount that eventually enters the general circulation depends on which route of delivery is used.

Pregnenolone taken orally first travels to the liver, which metabolizes it into other hormones. As a result, the amount of pregnenolone in circulation will be less than what was consumed. In contrast, micro-nized pregnenolone — in the form of tiny particles, taken as a capsule — is absorbed from the intestines directly into the lymphatic system, with most of it initially bypassing the liver. Another way to bypass the liver is by taking a sublingual tablet, which is absorbed through the tissue under the tongue. There is a spray, a chewing gum, and a liquid — all of which can deliver pregnenolone through the mouth — as well as a topical cream.

In retail stores, pregnenolone is available in capsule form in various dosages, including 10, 15, 25, 30, and 50 mg. It can also be found in combination with DHEA, vitamin C, vitamin E, and herbs such as ginkgo biloba. Compounding pharmacies working with physicians can prepare pregnenolone in doses from 2 to 100 mg. These pharmacies offer pregnenolone as a pill, a sublingual tablet, a cream, and a micronized capsule. Different delivery systems produce markedly different rates of assimilation and absorption. Be careful not to overdose if you switch from one method to another. Also, most dosages you will read about are based on pregnenolone in capsule form. Use the information below as a guideline for using a different delivery system. This information was supplied by VitalSource Nutrition.

Capsules

The assimilation and absorption rate is between 30 and 50 percent, because the pregnenolone is first processed through the liver before going into the bloodstream. Higher absorption rates may be attained by opening a capsule and releasing the contents under the tongue; hold this for a minute or two before swallowing.

Liquid Sublinguals

Assimilation and absorption rates run as high as 90 to 95 percent. This is because these are held under the tongue and the absorption is directly into the bloodstream, avoiding the liver. Sublinguals usually provide 5 mg of pregnenolone per drop, while liposome sprays usually contain 7.5 mg per spray.

Creams

The assimilation and absorption rate is between 50 and 85 percent. Absorption is also directly into the bloodstream, again avoiding the liver. The absorption rate depends on the quality of the cream, what carriers are present, where on the body the cream is applied (areas where skin is thinner or areas of fatty tissue), the cleanliness of the skin, and the humidity.

When pregnenolone is used for hormone replacement therapy, the dosage depends largely on age. In general, any usage of pregnenolone supplementation should begin at the lower end of the dosage range.

The range of dosages for women in their 40's is 5-10 mg, taken in the morning. For postmenopausal women, dosages range from 10-15 mg, taken in the morning, before or with breakfast. Women over 65 may need from 10-20 mg daily, taken in the morning. Do not take it in the evening, as it can increase your level of alertness and interfere with sleep.

If you are also taking progesterone as part of your hormone replacement program, the dosage may need to be reduced. Pregnenolone converted into progesterone adds to the overall supply of the body.

When pregnenolone is used to treat chronic health problems such as rheumatoid arthritis, effective dosages used in studies range from 100-200 mg. However, a dosage this high should be taken only under the supervision of a physician.

Side Effects

While animal and human studies have shown that pregnenolone is non-toxic, this powerful hormone should be used carefully, preferably under the supervision of a health care professional. There has been no formal assessment of its safety when used for years, and research on its side effects is only in the early stages. For instance, it is not known with certainty whether it is safe to allow pregnenolone to enter the general circulation without first passing through the liver, where it can be partially broken down.

If you are taking more pregnenolone than your system can handle, side effects such as irritability, anxiety, and anger may be experienced. Although there are no studies available, physicians who prescribe hormones suggest that pregnenolone and DHEA be taken in the morning, as the body appears to have its highest concentrations of these hormones at that time. If, however, pregnenolone is taken later in the day, it can cause overactivity and heightened alertness in sensitive individuals and may prevent them from falling asleep.

If you are taking any prescription or over-the-counter drugs, you should check with your physician for any possible negative interactions or dosage changes.

A Caution on Taking Pregnenolone

Individuals under 40, who normally produce ample levels of sex hormones, should not take pregnenolone. It is also not recommended during pregnancy, for people with cardiac problems, or for those who are taking multiple medications.

If you are using conventional HRT, you must consult with your prescribing physician before supplementing with pregnenolone, as it may affect the HRT dosages. Pregnenolone is a powerful hormone and should be treated as such.

Summary

Maintaining optimum pregnenolone levels not only improves the production and balance of all your sex hormones, but also improves your mental, emotional, and physical health. By following the program I've outlined in these two chapters, you can maintain proper overall hormone balance for years to come.

1. Maintain pregnenolone production at the central nervous system level with 5-HTP and tyrosine, as well as other supportive nutrients.

2. Support pregnenolone production in the adrenals and ovaries with glandulars, beta carotene, vitamin C, vitamin B5, zinc, and magnesium.

3. Support adrenal health with herbs such as Rhodiola rosea, Panax ginseng, and Siberian ginseng.

4. Use biochemically identical natural pregnen-olone.

About Susan M. Lark, M.D.

Dr. Susan Lark is one of the foremost authorities in the fields of women's health care and alternative medicine. Dr. Lark has successfully treated many thousands of women emphasizing holistic health and complementary medicine in her clinical practice. Her mission is to provide women with unique, safe and effective alternative therapies to greatly enhance their health and well-being.

A graduate of Northwestern University Feinberg School of Medicine, she has served on the clinical faculty of Stanford University Medical School, and taught in their Division of Family and Community Medicine.

Dr. Lark is a distinguished clinician, author, lecturer and innovative product developer. She has been an innovator in the use of self-care treatments such as diet, nutrition, exercise and stress management techniques in the field of women's health. She is the author of many best-selling books on women's health. Her signature line of nutritional supplements and skin care products are available through healthydirections.com.

One of the most widely referenced physicians on the Internet, Dr. Lark has appeared on numerous radio and television shows, and has been featured in many magazines and newspapers.

She has also served as a consultant to major corporations, including the Kellogg Company and Weider Nutrition International, and was spokesperson for The Gillette Company Women's Cancer Connection.

Dr. Lark can be contacted at (650) 561-9978 to make an appointment for a consultation.

Dr. Susan's Solutions
Health Library For Women

The following books are available from iTunes, Amazon.com, Amazon Kindle, Womens Wellness Publishing and other major booksellers. Dr. Susan is frequently adding new books to her health library.

Women's Health Issues

Dr. Susan's Solutions: Heal Endometriosis

Dr. Susan's Solutions: Healthy Heart and Blood Pressure

Dr. Susan's Solutions: Healthy Menopause

Dr. Susan's Solutions: The Anemia Cure

Dr. Susan's Solutions: The Bladder Infection Cure

Dr. Susan's Solutions: The Candida-Yeast Infection Cure

Dr. Susan's Solutions: The Chronic Fatigue Cure

Dr. Susan's Solutions: The Cold and Flu Cure

Dr. Susan's Solutions: The Fibroid Tumor Cure

Dr. Susan's Solutions: The Irregular Menstruation Cure

Dr. Susan's Solutions: The Menstrual Cramp Cure

Dr. Susan's Solutions: The PMS Cure

Emotional and Spiritual Balance

Breathing Meditations for Healing, Peace and Joy

Dr. Susan's Solutions: The Anxiety and Stress Cure

Women's Hormones

Dr. Susan's Solutions: DHEA
Dr. Susan's Solutions: Pregnenolone
Dr. Susan's Solutions: Progesterone
Dr. Susan's Solutions: Testosterone
Healthy, Natural Estrogens for Menopause

Diet and Nutrition

Dr. Susan Lark's Healing Herbs for Women
Dr. Susan Lark's Complete Guide to Detoxification
Enzymes: The Missing Link to Health
Healthy Diet and Nutrition for Women: The
Complete Guide
Renew Yourself Through Juice Fasting and
Detoxification Diets

Energy Therapies and Anti-Aging

Acupressure for Women: Relieve Symptoms of
Dozens of Health Issues Through Pressure Points

Exercise and Flexibility

Stretching and Flexibility for Women
Stretching Programs for Women's Health Issues

About Womens Wellness Publishing

"Bringing Radiant Health and Wellness to Women"

Womens Wellness Publishing was founded to make a positive difference in the lives of women and their families. We are the premier publisher of print and eBooks focused on women's health and wellness. We are committed to publishing the finest quality and most comprehensive line of books that covers every area that a woman needs to create vibrant health and a joyful, fulfilling life.

Our books are written and created by the top health and wellness experts who share with you, our readers, their wisdom and extensive experience successfully treating many thousands of patients.

We encourage you to browse through our online bookstore; new books are frequently being added to womenswellnesspublishing.com. Visit our Lifestyle Center and Customer Bonus Center for more exciting and helpful health and wellness information and resources.

Follow us on Facebook for the latest health tips, recipes, and all natural solutions to many women's health issues (facebook.com/wwpublishing).

We would enjoy hearing from you! Please share your success stories, comments and requests for new topics at yourstory@wwpublishing.com.

About Our Associate Program

We invite you to become part of the Womens Wellness Publishing Community through our Associate Program. You will have the opportunity to earn generous commissions on sales that you create through your blog, social network, support groups, community groups, school & alumni groups, friends, family or other networks.

To join the Associate Program, go to our website, womenswellnesspublishing.com, and click "Become an Associate"

We support your sales and marketing efforts by offering you and your customers:

- Free support materials with updates on all of our new book releases, promotions, and bonuses for you and your customers
- Free audio downloads, booklets, and guides
- Special discounts and sales promotions

27944203R00040

Made in the USA
Lexington, KY
30 November 2013